Blood Group Diet

Eating Right for Your Blood Group 101

By Cathy Wilson

ISBN-13:
978-1493766062

ISBN-10:
1493766066

First Printing, 2013

Printed in the United States of America

Income Disclaimer

This book contains business strategies, marketing methods and other business advice that, regardless of my own results and experience, may not produce the same results (or any results) for you. I make absolutely no guarantee, expressed or implied, that by following the advice below you will make any money or improve current profits, as there are several factors and variables that come into play regarding any given business.

Primarily, results will depend on the nature of the product or business model, the conditions of the marketplace, the experience of the individual, and situations and elements that are beyond your control.

As with any business endeavor, you assume all risk related to investment and money based on your own discretion and at your own potential expense.

Liability Disclaimer

By reading this book, you assume all risks associated with using the advice given below, with a full understanding that you, solely, are responsible for anything that may occur as a result of putting this information into action in any way, and regardless of your interpretation of the advice.

You further agree that our company cannot be held responsible in any way for the success or failure of your business as a result of the information presented in this book. It is your responsibility to conduct your own due diligence regarding the safe and successful operation of your business if you intend to apply any of our information in any way to your business operations.

Terms of Use

You are given a non-transferable, “personal use” license to this book. You cannot distribute it or share it with other individuals.

Also, there are no resale rights or private label rights granted when purchasing this book. In other words, it's for your own personal use only.

Blood Group Diet

Eating Right for Your Blood Group 101

By Cathy Wilson

Table of Contents

Introduction

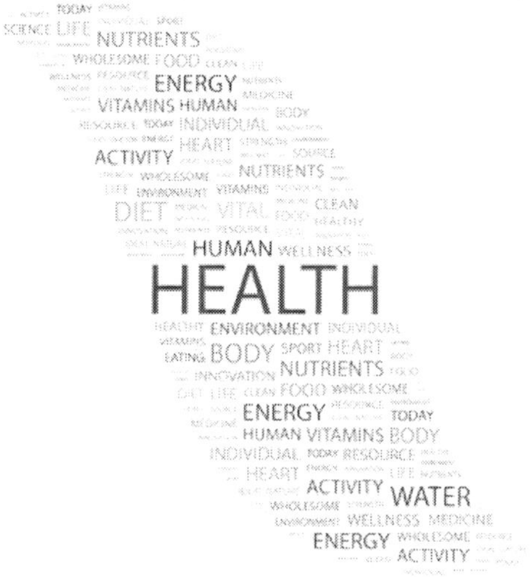

* The Benefits of Eating "Right" for your Blood Type are crystal clear: increased energy, diminishing food tolerances, disease prevention, reducing or eliminating symptoms of disease and Illness, increasing cognitive capacity, zapping fat, and that's just a start!

The Purpose? Eating "right" for your blood type is focused on helping people stay healthy, live a longer and more fulfilling life, zap disease inducing free radicals, reach and attain their ideal weight for life, which of course sounds appealing to us all.

The basic theory is that each blood type or group affects the digestive system a little differently. So if you can learn to get your nutrition from the foods that work best with your blood type and individual body systems, then your body is going to work more efficiently and effectively as a whole; mind, body and soul.

And by steering clear of foods that don't sit well in accordance to your blood type, you'll avoid minor nuisances and deter the development of life-threatening conditions that occur over time. This evolutionary theory of eating for your blood type stems further still to conclude specific exercising that is most beneficial to particular blood types. But we are going to focus on "food" angle for now.

Many are attracted to this diet because they don't have to fret about the headache of tracking fat and calories, which you have to admit can really be a pain in the rear.

The blood type diet also works better if you either live on your own or the people in the household all have the same blood type. This definitely makes "Eating Right For Your Blood Group" a heck of a lot easier to apply. I'm not going to promise you this diet is the "end-all-be-all" of health and wellness because that would just be yanking your chain. But if you can learn one or two positive health benefits through the "Blood Group Diet," that are going to help deter disease, help you look younger, live longer and have a more balanced mental capacity, isn't it worth your while? Just keep that thought in mind as you learn the basics of "Eating Right For Your Blood Group."

Blood Examined in Basic

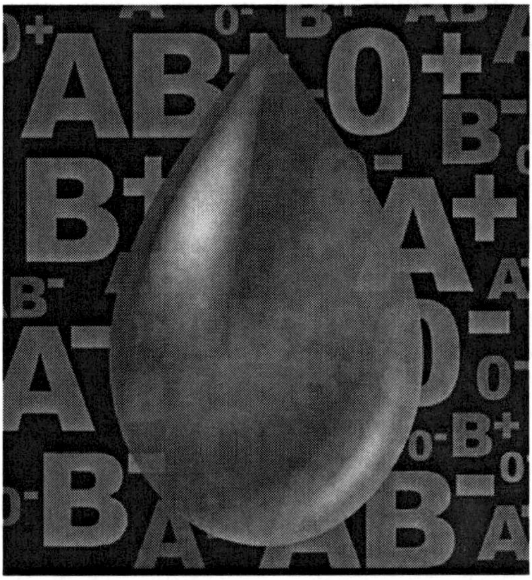

What is Blood?

Defined, blood is the bodily fluid that transports essential substances including oxygen and vital nutrients to the cells of the body, while taking metabolic waste products of toxins and ridding the body of them.

Blood circulates through your body with the help of your heart in a pumping, contracting action. In humans the blood is made of blood cells that are encompassed by blood plasma. Plasma is mainly used for the vehicle for excretory product. Plasma makes up about 55% of blood fluid, which is mainly composed of water. It also contains glucose, minerals, hormones, CO_2, proteins and blood cells.

Here are the different types of blood just to give you a solid base from which to start.

* Occult Blood is only detectable by chemical testing because it's in such tiny amounts.
* Arterial Blood essentially is blood with oxygen and is found in your veins, left changes in the heart and your arteries.
* Whole blood hasn't had anything removed from it.
* Citrated blood has been treated with citric acid or sodium citrate so it doesn't get thick and coagulated.
* Pre-donated Autologous blood is donated blood that may be used for a surgical procedure.
* Cord blood is found in the umbilical cord of a newborn infant, the lifeline between mother and baby.
* Venous blood is where oxygen is given up and blood is being carried away from the tissues of your body.

So I think you've got a pretty good idea of what blood is and now we're going to shift gears and look into the different types of blood. If you don't know your blood type a simple blood test at your doctors will tell you. This is very important to know for the sake of good health and good eating!

Blood Types Explained

Your blood type is something you are stuck with for life. It's not something you could even change if you wanted to. There are advantages and disadvantages to each of the 4 blood types; A, AB, B, and O. It's always best to start from the bottom and work your way up. So we're going to start by looking at the basic concepts of each of the different blood types in order to get warmed up.

The basic elements in all blood types are essentially the same, however not all blood is the same. You may be surprised to know there are actually eight different well known blood types, recognized by the amount of specific antigens, which are specific substances that will catalyze a reaction to a foreign substance in the body. There are antigens that will cause a person's blood to initiate an attack on the transfused blood and this makes blood-typing prior to a transfusion very important.

FACT - The four main blood groups, A, AB, B and O, are recognized by the presence or absence of two specific antigens, A and B, on the top or surface of the blood cell.

A - This group has the A antigen on the surface, with the antibody B in the plasma.
A + is the second most common blood type in Caucasians and it's fairly popular with all other ethnicities. However it's safe to say the A - is much less popular across the board.

B - This group has the B antigen on the surface of the red blood cells, with antibody A in the plasma. B+ is very rare in general but B - is extremely rare. In fact it's found in only 2% of Caucasians.

AB - A and B antigens for this group are present on the surface of the blood cell, with neither antibody A or B in the plasma. AB is the rarest blood group, with AB - found in less than 1% of Caucasians.

O - With this group you have neither antigen A or B on the surface, and both antibodies A and B are found in the plasma. O + is the most common blood type in all ethnicities. However O - is found in only 8% of Caucasians.

Your blood type is determined by genetics, derived from the blood groups of your parents.

BLOOD DONOR KNOWLEDGE FOR THOUGHT

When donating blood there are specific ways the blood must be matched in order to have a successful transfusion

* The O group is able to donate RBC to any person, known as the universal donor.
* The A group is able to donate red blood cells to anyone with A or AB blood group.
* The B group has the ability to donate RBC to the B and AB group.
* The group AB can give to other abs, and can also receive from any blood group.

SPECIAL NOTE - There is a third antigen besides A and B and that's the RH factor. It can be either negative or positive. RH - blood can be administered to RH - people and RH + or - can be given to RH + people.

Type O negative is the universal donor blood and AB positive is the universal plasma donor.

My Thinking . . .

I understand the science behind blood can get a touch complex,but having the necessary understanding behind what blood is and how it is composed is important in making the connection because blood and nutrition. So don't worry too much about the technical, what's im-

portant is that you have a basic understanding from which to build and apply new information.

Nutrition and Blood Type Basics Teaser

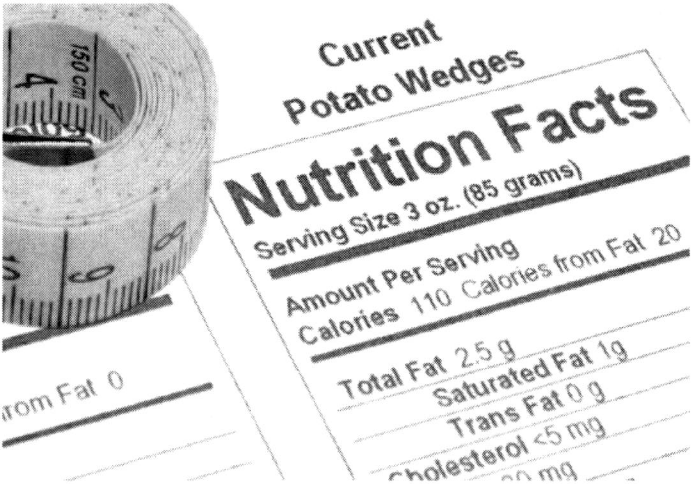

The idea here is that your specific blood type is suggestive of the prehistoric ancestry you come from, which give clues as to what particular foods your digestive system tolerates and doesn't. If we switch our thinking to genetics, group O type blood is the eldest of the four main groups.

So what has this got to do with the food you eat?

Well it means people with this genetically older blood type need to eat meat every day because the earliest people were hunters and gatherers that lived off the land, with a free - range game as their main source of nutrition. This is how they are to survive. Protein was vital to their existence.

Experts believe individuals with group A blood are linked to ancient agrarian roots, implying their diet should follow vegetarian. Interesting don't you think? And I'm not going to mislead you here because there is controversy in this genetic theory of blood type and diet. Although one constant among all professionals is the type of blood you have does in fact influence your health. To what degree is where the controversy begins, hence we begin.

Blood Group Diet History/Disease

The blood type diet is an eating strategy whereby one eats specific foods depending on their genetic blood group, which is absolute. This evolutionary based diet was created by Peter D'Adamo, claiming that the ABO blood type is critical in dictating what foods are best for each different blood group. He uses the study results of various accredited glycobiologists and biochemists to stamp validity of his claims.

The basis of his D'Adamo's claim is that your blood type is vital in seeing the difference between "self" and "non-self." The historical facts of his theory are that lectins which are found in food, react differently depending on your blood group. Particularly with the antigens and this deems specific foods more tolerable than others. Further still, some lectins are harmful. Lectins are proteins that bind with carbohydrates that are in tune with sugar molecules, scientifically speaking.

By eating certain foods with specific blood groups you will theoretically avoid or at least minimize harmful lectin reactions. D'Adamo uses the ABO classification system and various classification and surface tissue antigens to support his theories.

D'Adamo had a partner is crime from which he advanced the blood type diet from William Boyd. In the 50s body released a book which deduced through the analysis genetically of blood groups, humans can be divided into populations in accordance to their alleles or genes. D'Adamo took these findings and grouped the in blood types with specific diet allocated to each.

* O Blood - Hunter

The belief is this is the oldest blood group, over 30,000 years old and requires higher protein foods. With regards to disease, group O is more likely to suffer from hay fever, asthma and various other allergies. Arthritis is also an issue with O blood type because their immune systems have issues tolerating the environment. Grain foods especially will trigger inflammation of the joints.

* A Blood - Cultivator

Historically stemming from approximately 20,000 years ago with the beginning of agricultural focus. The eating here should be vegetarian focused with no red meat. With diseases, this blood group is at higher risk for developing diabetes, along with a higher rate of cancer with a lower chance of survival.

* B Blood - Nomad

Historically arriving 10,000 years ago this grouping attunes to a strong immune system and tolerable digestive system, developing in the Himalayan Highlands which is not a part of India and Pakistan. It's believed the group B blood type could have been altered initially because of drastic climatic changes. This blood type is often sensitive to balance between vegetation and animals.

Higher than normal cortisol levels are often produced which makes optimal health a challenge. The result is often inflammation, slow growth, viruses that linger and a higher susceptibility to immune system disease. And because of the whacky cortisol levels group B individuals are often overwhelmed easily with stress.

The suggested eating here is lots of dairy products. With disease, this group is highly resistant to allergies, but we are at increased susceptibility to autoimmune issues like lupus, chronic fatigue, and MS, as well as a higher risk of diabetes.

RED FLAG - This issue with this specific theory is the majority of Asians are B group blood and are often lactose intolerant because their body is unable to break down milk products. You can see here a little bit of controversy is brewing.

* AB Blood - Enigma

This was thought to be the newest blood type arriving just 1,000 years ago. This group is seen as between group A and B. In disease, group AB has a few issues with asthma and allergies, although low iron (anemia), cardiovascular disease and cancer are higher risk. AB blood type can also have one of the highest risks of cancer with poorest survival rate.

My Thinking . . .

This theory seems to make sense on the surface. There are solid correlations scientifically linked or not. Take this base blood group knowledge, its evolutionary history and suggested implications, store them somewhere in thoughts and open your mind to a few new concepts that will help you make better food choices for your body.

Better Food Choices for Your Blood Type

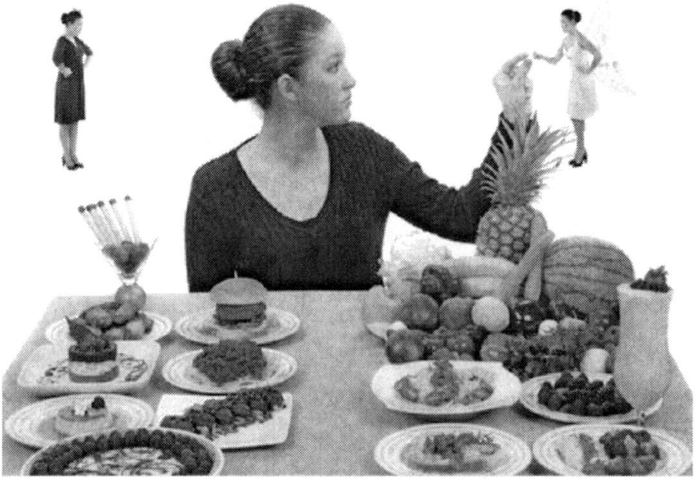

Eating Tips Blood Type A

Just think vegetarian eating here. Symbolic of the loss of some of the savagery of the hunter and the transition into natural farming practices. This diet is centered on healthy whole grains, organic vegetables, and soy. The belief is the digestive tract does well with a fibrous diet full of healthy vitamins and essential minerals, minus the stress on the body breaking down meat protein.

Contrary to many misconceptions you can get all the nutrients required for optimal health from a vegan diet.

Understanding meat is the easiest way to get the complete protein that's required for numerous bodily functions, including muscle building and brain function.

Quinoa is one of the only non-meat complete proteins and is excellent for someone with type A blood. Another strategy to get enough digestible protein without eating meat is to combine specific vegetables to equal complete protein. So some effort is required initially but then it should be smooth sailing.

With regards to exercising, according to the "Eating for your Blood Type Diet," group A blood type is naturally in tune with gentle exercising. Most yoga's, walking, light jogging and biking, strength training and light weights are great options.

Expected Health Issues Extended

* Lower levels natural stomach acid
* Temper-mental digestive system
* Cancer and diabetes
* Cardiovascular disease
* Infections and an overproduction of mucus

Description Body Type and Characteristics

* Particularly negative towards B blood type people
* Often thin, smart and emotional
* Stimulated by conversation and debate
* Extreme emotionally (highs/lows)

General Guidelines

* Does well eating tofu, fruit, beans and legumes, veggies and healthy whole grains
* Stay away from most meat

* Don't eat any dairy
* Try not to eat processed foods
* Fish, soy and some vegetables will help you get adequate protein
* Stay clear of wheat, will trigger mucus increase
* Avoid dairy, meat, lima and kidney beans to improve energy levels and stay lean
* Deal with stress by doing calming and relaxing exercises

Note: With this blood type eating ideology the body functions optimally with some alkalinity. It's important natural foods are consumed and processed, pre-packaged and frozen foods are avoided. This is mainly because they have various chemicals and additives that are going to interfere with the running of the body as a whole. Make a habit of using foods nature provides that are whole and natural, without spices. Just think apples, bananas, broccoli, spinach and quinoa.

Eating Tips Blood Type B

According to the blood diet theory, this blood type is more tolerant in general. So, blood type B people are encouraged to eat lean meat, low fat dairy and healthy fresh produce. It's a system that is evolutionarily conditioned to process and digest most foods with optimum effectiveness.

According to evolution individuals with blood type B can digest most foods easily.

* digestive systems that are highly tolerant
* dairy products are broken down easily
* wheat products with gluten are the difficult to digest

Food items to stay away from are:

* corn
* lentils
* wheat
* peanuts
* chicken
* sesame seeds
* buckwheat

Foods to Help Encourage Weight Loss

* soy
* flax seed oil and olive oil in moderation
* oat bran and oatmeal
* green veggies
* lower fat dairy and eggs
* red meats including rabbit, liver, mutton, pheasant and turkey
* salmon, flounder, halibut and sole
* puffed rice and rice bran

Type B's tend to have issues with when products, causing a natural blood sugar drop and low blood sugar or hypoglycemia. Similar to what you experience after coming down from a simple sugar junky sugar rush.

Other foods to avoid are:

- lentils, shellfish, tomatoes, artichokes, pumpkin, radishes, coconut, rhubarb, allspice, almond extract, cinnamon, cornstarch, corn syrup, gelatin, pepper, ketchup, liquor, soda, barley, cornflakes, cream of wheat, shredded wheat, multi-grain, wheat germ, canola oil, sunflower oil, safflower oil and cottonseed oil.

Expected Health Issues

* Does tend to develop disorders of the immune system
* Arthritis with swelling
* Low Iron and not because of no meat
* Neurological disorders

Body Type and Characteristics

* Poor food choices results in blood sugar drop after meals
* Can have issues with blood A group people
* Friendly nature, nurturing
* Depends of close relationships in general
* Could have reproductive issues

General Guidelines

* Most compatible blood groups that do well with lean meats and fish, fresh vegetables and dairy products
* DO NOT eat tomatoes, olives, chicken, rye, corn, wheat, buckwheat
* High calorie is okay
* Creativity works to relieve stress
* Mental and physical activity is required to stay sharp and lean. A balance is required.

Eating Tips Blood Type AB

Did you know that less than five percent of the global population has group AB blood?

Rare and very precious is this AB blood type. According to the Blood Type Diet it has been around for only about a thousand years. It makes sense that most foods on the "don't eat" list for type A and B blood groups are also in place for type ABs, with the exception of tomatoes.

With group AB they seem to have the ability to tolerate tomato lectins with no issue. AB also doesn't have adequate amounts of stomach acid to easily break down an-animal protein, including chicken, beef and fish. Now this doesn't mean you shouldn't have ANY animal protein, just keep it to a minimum. What helps with this is taking bromelain, which is a digestive enzyme from pineapples that will naturally help with breaking down the protein so your body can use it.

If you are looking to gain weight these are great nutrition options.

* lima and kidney beans
* red meat
* various seeds and corn
* wheat and buckwheat

Losing weight for blood group AB foods are:

* pineapple
* spirulina and sea kelp
* green veggies and tofu
* low-fat dairy products
* seafood
* tofu

Other Meat to Avoid

- Bacon, beef, buffalo, ground beef, chicken, venison, pork, veal

Fruits to Steer Around

- Oranges, mangoes, coconuts, bananas, guava, pomegranates, star fruit, rhubarb, pears (prickly)

Seafood to Avoid

- Turtle, bass, shrimp, sole, frog, haddock, halibut, beluga, anchovies, clams, conch, barracuda, crayfish, flounder, eel, lox, oysters, octopus, pickled herring

Veggies to Sidestep

- Radishes, sprouts, peppers, black olives, artichokes, corn, lima beans, avocado

Dairy Products to Stay Away From

- Sherbet, full fat milk, cheese (American, Brie, Blue, Parmesan, provolone), ice cream, buttermilk, butter

Pastas, Grains and Cereals to Avoid

- Buckwheat noodles, barley flour, artichoke pasta, buckwheat flour, corn muffins, cornmeal, cornflakes, kasha and kamut

Oils to Avoid

- Sesame, safflower, cottonseed, corn, peanut

Legumes/Beans to Stay away From

-Lima, kidney, black-eyes peas, azuki black, garbanzo, Vicia faba

Seeds/Nuts to Avoid

- Sunflower, sesame, poppy, and pumpkin seeds, tahini, sunflower butter

Expected Health Issues

* Very little stomach acid
* Too much mucus
* Asthma
* Lots of infections

Body Type and Characteristics

* Reflective thinking yet pessimistic
* Keeps stresses hidden
* Prefers to live on cloud nine
* Generally gets along with just about anyone by choice
* Analyzes too much, even loses sleep over it

General Guidelines

* Fish, tofu and vegetables are best
* Lots of different foods work if they are kept in moderation
* Stay away from simple sugars, tomatoes, corn, buckwheat
* To lose weight and stay energetic don't eat red meat, corn, seeds, wheat, kidney and lima beans
* Spirituality and creativity is best for stress

Eating Tips Blood Type O

"O" stands for old here, where your digestive system has the memories engrained from the ancient days past, theoretically. Blood O type people will benefit from plenty of lean meat in their diet because that's what history dictates. The first people on earth were thought to be hunters and gatherers, whereby the majority of their dietary needs were met through various game meats.

Good choices are lean poultry, meats and fish. Grains both complex and simple should be consumed sporadically. The same goes for legumes and breads. When it comes to exercise just think about a hungry tiger chasing a poor hunter that was thrown from his horse. Rigorous exercise is natural and most beneficial for O blood candidates under this interesting diet regimen.

Expected Health Issues

* Tiredness/fatigue
* Leans towards elevated blood pressure
* Leans towards elevated cholesterol
* Bowel issues
* Thyroid weakness caused by adrenal weakness
* Excess stomach acid which increases ulcer risk
* Potential blood clotting issues because of thin blood

Body Type and Characteristics

* Tough gaining weight
* Great physical strength
* Determined, works hard
* Physical activity is natural
* Thinks caffeine/coffee improves performance
* Enjoys meat and potatoes
* Weak liver triggers quick anger
* Loves to give to everyone, may have issues with blood group A and B
* Very strong beliefs/passion

General Guidelines

* Better eating smaller portions
* Does well on veggies and lean meats
* Steer clear of breads and pasta (carbs), simple sugars, dairy, grains
* Needs "clean" eating to ensure maximized metabolism, avoiding grains to gain energy and stay lean

* Hardcore intense exercise works best

Foods to Eat

Meats - fish, beef, veal, venison, mutton, lamb

Fats and Oils - olive oil and flaxseed oil (monounsaturated oils preferred)

Seeds/Nuts - walnuts, pumpkin

Legumes/Beans - pinto, black-eyed pea, aduke, azuki

Whole Grains, Cereals, Pasta and Bread - Ezekiel and Essene bread in moderation

Vegetables - sweet potato, artichoke, chicory, broccoli, beet, escarole, collard, dandelion, leek, kale, horseradish, kohlrabi, okra, romaine lettuce, red pepper, parsnips, parsley, onions, dandelion, pumpkin, seaweed, turnips, Swiss chard

Fruit - Prunes, cherries, plums, figs

Spices - Curry, carob, turmeric, kelp, dulse, Cayenne pepper, parsley

IMPORTANT NOTE: Fresh organic vegetables are first choice, then frozen and canned.

Foods to Stay Away From

Meats - pig meat, barracuda, goose, lox, octopus, herring, conch, caviar, catfish

Dairy Products and Eggs - If used in all, an digestive enzyme should also be taken

Fats and Oils - peanut, corn and safflower

Seeds/Nuts - peanuts, poppy seed, litchi, brazil, cashew, pistachio

Legumes/Beans - red, green, tamarind, navy, kidney, domestic, copper

Whole grains, cereals, pasta and bread - sprouts, semolina, white and wheat flour, corn, bulgur, farina, familia, graham, oat, pumpernickel, gluten, matzos, soba, spinach

Vegetables - cabbage, avocado, corn, mushrooms, eggplant, mustard greens, potato (red/white), cauliflower, sprouts

JUICE NOTE: Vegetable juice is the best choice to help stay away from sweeteners and balance your alkaline/acid levels. Having a state with slight acidity is advantageous.

My Thinking . . .

Use this information to help guide you in making better decisions for your body. Hopefully you can make the logical connections as to why you do well with certain foods and others not so well. Don't be afraid to try something new and make sure you are adding to your nutritional knowledge base each day.

By making small adjustments that you can learn to accept and eventually transform into your new "normal," you are setting yourself up for success. It seems pretty obvious there is a connection between blood type and nutrition. Maybe we don't need to focus so much on ex-

actly what this connection is, but rather take the expert information gathered and just apply it as we see fit? It's something to think about.

Blood Type and Personality

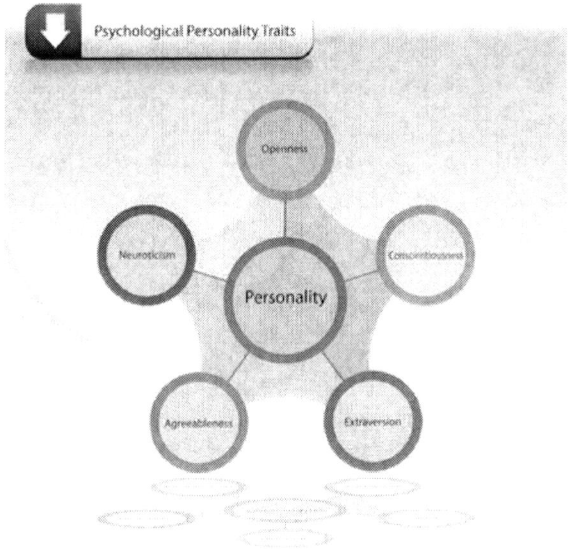

The evolutionary theory with eating for your blood type is that your personality is interconnected on some level. The argument here between experts, scientists and qualified professionals is first if there is enough scientific evidence to back this claim up and secondly, to what degree is it considered relevant. I won't bore you with the heated battle back and forth. What I find interesting here is there seems to be a pattern and common traits that suggest connection between your birth blood and how you act and present yourself.

I'll start saying this theory is especially popular in Japan. That being said, in the early 1900s Germans found that specific races had specific blood types, for the most part anyway. Of course you understand there are always exceptions to the rules and this is a very broad based theory. You do have to start somewhere right?

This theory of interlinking blood type with personality died down and re-emerged about twenty-five years later with a study completed in Tokyo at a teaching school. A detailed study between blood type and temperament was conducted. Suffice to say there wasn't enough scientific evidence for the results to fly and merit was lost. Although this was enough to keep the interest of the world peaked and searching for solid evidence.

In the early 70's another book by Masahiko about "Understanding Affinity with Relation to Blood Type" was released. Again no scientific backing but this fueled the fire to learn more. Japan believed in it and took it to the bank.

In Japanese culture they use blood type to pick partner matches on dating sites and celebrities will often include their blood type in general conversation. It's important to them, although this may seem a touch weird for most Westerners. Could you imagine asking your date what blood type they are?

On this unproven scientific theory, that specific blood type reflects personality, here are the generalizations.

O TYPE

- Outgoing, social
- Initiators that like to get the party started
- Often don't complete the task at hand

- Self-confident in general
- Love being the center of attention
- Popular, creative
- "No-fear" attitude
- Trendsetters
- Passionate about what they love
- Energetic
- Extroverted

A TYPE

- Calm, peaceful
- Perfectionist
- Internal anxiety (self-manifested)
- Most artistic
- Trustworthy, sensitive
- Worrisome, quiet
- Sensitive to emotions
- Organized, serious

B TYPE

- Goal focused
- Strong thinking
- Determined
- Finished what they started well
- Own unique way of life
- Moodiness and insensitive at times
- Set minds, reaches goals they care about
- Practical, hardworking
- Laid back, casual

AB TYPE

- Split between A and B
- Variety
- Outgoing and timid

- Responsible but easily overwhelmed
- Helpful, trusting
- Forgives others
- Tough on self
- Rare

MATCHING BLOOD TYPE AND PERSONALITY

A~Matches with A and B
B~Matches with B and AB
AB~Matches with AB, B, A and O
O~Matches with O or AB

My Thinking . . .

These findings between blood type and personalities really are quite neat. Scientific proof or not I can definitely see connections and pretty solid ones at that. One more piece of information that just might save you some future heartaches or relationship stress if you can apply it in moderation. Just a thought . . .

Blood Type and Digestion

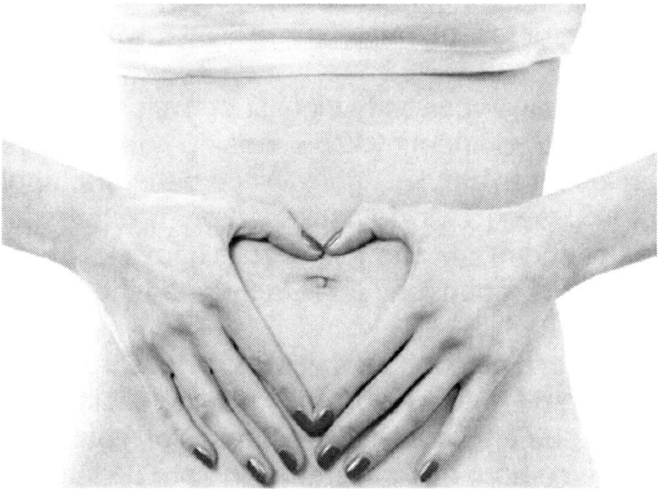

Another linked connection with blood and diet and health is with digestion. The process in which your body takes fuel (food) and breaks it down into energy your body can use to keep your internal systems smiling. Recognizing if your body wasn't able to digest you wouldn't be going anywhere. How effectively your body breaks food down, absorbs and discards waste is directly reflective of your overall health, including how you look, feel and function.

For instance, if you are eating processed foods loaded with harmful additives and preservatives that build up in your system because your body can't metabolize or break them down, you are going to develop health issues in time. To start, you're likely to feel sluggish, lack energy, have skin issues, unexplained aches and pains, and you probably battle with your weight. By making better food choices that your body can digest better you're going to look and feel better and your health will start looking brighter. That's just a very general idea just to get us started.

In basic, the theory here is each blood type has a different ability to digest proteins.

* Eating proteins your body digests or metabolizes easily will help keep you healthy. So choosing natural fruits and vegetables for example is going to be better metabolized than a processed Twinkie packaged on the shelf, full of all sorts of chemicals and toxins your body can't break down. Doesn't mean they don't taste good though.

* Diseases can be avoided if your body absorbs specific nutrients from foods. The trick is knowing exactly how much of a nutrient your body absorbs. You could be eating oranges galore and assuming you are getting lots of vitamin C for instance. But if you have a condition that doesn't allow your body to soak up the vitamin you can unknowingly be denying your body what it needs.

When we're looking at digestion and different blood groups it's important to know the basic of antigens and lectins

Lectins are the proteins in food.
Antigens are what blocks part of the food so the body can't digest it. In other words antigens interfere with digestion. They're the "bad" guys.

So the thought is that each blood group has its own mechanisms of digestion and their own gastrointestinal tract that is projected for specific kinds of food. Getting the "right" foods or fuel allows the digestive system to get adequate nutrients to balance good health.

DIGESTION - shred or chew food - saliva mixes with enzymes - splits sugars and starch and waste

DIGESTION of BLOOD TYPE A and AB

- There's always a shortage of stomach acid
- This causes natural overgrowth of bacteria in the upper intestine and stomach which is often chronic

DIGESTION OF BLOOD TYPE A

- Common issues are inactive pepsin and hardly any split of proteins
- Blood type A seems to always have issues with digestion
- Theory is the A antigen in the juice of the stomach connects with the pepsin and actually stops the spitting of protein, which of course is essential in digestion

Let's look at the chemical of digestion in your intestine.

Intestine - considering alkaline phosphatase for meat breakdown

The amount of alkaline phosphatase is usually excellent for blood type B and O and not very good with blood type A. In blood type O the intestine releases lots of the alkaline enzyme phosphatase. This splits the proteins of meat and fish really efficiently in use.

In blood type B alkaline phosphate is there but not as much as O. With blood type A it's scarcely there. Meaning a moderate amount of meat and meat products makes sense with type B blood and none with group A.

Further still, this alkaline enzyme splits cholesterol and the fat in food. So it makes sense the levels of cholesterol in type O and B are usually low. A and AB are stuck with lower levels of the enzyme so they tend to have issues with protein and higher cholesterol and fat levels in general. In black and white this means higher risk of heart attack and stroke.

The little bit of enzyme phosphatase type A has, is short circuited by its own A antigens. The bottom line is the A blood type isn't structured to break down lean meats.

DIGESTION OF BLOOD TYPE B

Type B blood group tends to have a sensitivity to food which interferes with achieving optimal health. It's issues with digesting foods including wheat, lentils, corn, tomatoes, sesame seeds and peanuts causes problems. Some of which are increased tiredness, swelling and hypoglycemia (drastic blood sugar level drops). Chicken is also another food that causes digestion issues because of large amounts of pectin in the muscle tissue. By eliminating these "interference" foods, blood type B individuals can lose weight and build strong and healthy bodies that will stand strong against the stress of time.

DIGESTION OF BLOOD TYPE O

As you may have expected, blood type O does well again here. The naturally high level of alkaline phosphate in their blood enables them to digest foods more effectively and efficiently, particularly meat, which is harder for other blood types to break down. The alkaline phosphatase enzyme not only looks favorably at breaking down fat but also looks good on calcium. The evidence this enzyme supports calcium absorption is that blood group O people have fewer fractures and a decreased amount of osteoporosis as a whole compared to other blood types.

The bottom line here is different blood types need different foods for optimal health and wellness. Varying proteins are broken down and utilized in different ways and at different rates in accordance with their blood types. If the "wrong" foods are eaten this can cause issues with digestion, the immune system and metabolism, the rate in which the body burns fuel.

* Numerous lectins prefer specific sugar compounds and match with specific blood groups. If the blood types and lectins don't fit together, the proteins can't be broken down or digested.

It's pretty tough to question the importance of blood types and the best foods to eat when you consider all this information, wouldn't you agree?

My Thinking . . .

You are what you are right? So why would you try and eat foods your body doesn't digest well? Assuming of course you know what foods these are. Listen to your body and use the diet for your blood type general thinking to help you figure out what suits your unique system best. Keep an open mind and don't be afraid to experiment. You don't have to battle your body when it comes to eating "right." Make sound decisions and listen to what your body is telling you. It will be surprising how easy it is to exist in harmony if that's what you truly want.

Blood Type ABO and Cancer Risk

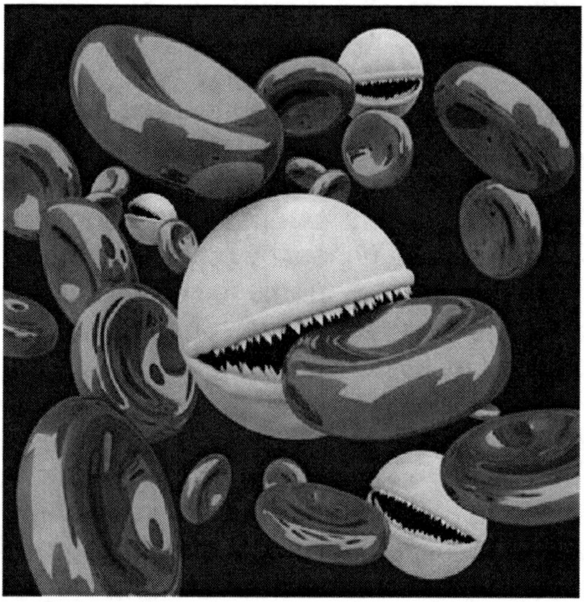

Cancer 101

Just hearing the word "cancer" is enough to make your heart skip a beat or two. Cancer is a disease that isn't new and knows no boundaries. The world has set out full force to battle and defeat this relentless and often inevitable death sentence. We have made huge progress in treating various cancers and prolonging life. The main interference has now been the steady increase in the number of overall cases. This world factor takes some of the wind out of our sails.

The following cancers are a sample few that has increased significantly over the past few years:

* Colon
* Breast
* Prostate
* Lung
* Rectal

Unfortunately experts agree this increase may be due to controllable lifestyle habits including smoking, exposure to environmental toxins, lack of exercise and unhealthy food choices, particularly increased ingestion of Trans Fats and dangerously unhealthy processed foods. There's also the payback for modern conveniences like cell phones and easily accessible drugs. Links to cancer are recognized as evidence mounts.

WHAT IS CANCER?

It's a basic term used for an inclusive group of more than 100 diseases identified by the out of control growth of abnormal cells that spreads quickly throughout the body. Each organ in your body is made of normal cells that will divide and create when needed. What happens is sometimes the body grows cells when they aren't needed and this forms masses called tumors. These tumors are either non-cancerous (benign), or cancerous (malignant).

What happens is cancerous tumors can invade other cells and even break off and filtrate through the blood or lymphatic system to poison other organs of the body. The spreading of cancer throughout the body is technically called metastasis.

The trigger of cancers is called carcinogens and can be for the environment, physical, biological or chemical. There are two different categories of carcinogens; Direct-Acting and Procarcinogens.

Direct Acting Carcinogens are carcinogenic by themselves.
Procacinogens must be transformed through your metabolic system into carcinogens.

It often takes years for carcinogens to develop and show face in a tumor. During this creation time the division of carcinogens can be summarized in two stages: initiation and promotion of tumor. In other words something initiates or triggers the tumor, like a chemical, physical or biological agent that damages the cell irreversibly. The promoter or fuel for the cell growth doesn't have to be carcinogenic in nature but it does promote continued growth of these "sick" cells. It's the anti-promoters that are often able to stop this abnormal cell division. Antioxidants are examples of anti-promoters, acting favorably to halt carcinogenic cells from subdividing. Fresh berries come to mind when loading your body with powerful disease fighting antioxidants.

Diet, genetics, gender, lifestyle and environmental factors are all considerations in the development of the initiator or carcinogenic cells in the first place. These factors also play a role in "if" these muted cells develop, at what pace, and if they will respond to treatment or not.

Cancer and Blood Type Explained

In the past there has been huge controversy of the studies involving cancer and blood type, namely because the studies conducted have been small and it really does seem tough to satisfy those that qualify "scientific validity." It is tough however to argue with results of base protein immune studies suggesting strongly that blood type antigens play a critical biological role, which is often not related to the RBC at all. Experts agree that IN GENERAL, cancers seem to be associated with type A, and a little less with B. Interesting generalization from the experts.

Breast Cancer

This is the most common cancer in women. Treatment options include:

- Lumpectomy surgery (remove a tumor and surrounding tissue)
- Mastectomy (remove whole breast)
- Radiation
- Chemotherapy
- Hormone blocking therapy

Usually a combined approach is used, depending on the situation. What often isn't mentioned with breast cancer is that susceptibility and outcome is influenced by blood type. Some experts even believe that cancers are indeed predictable with regards to blood types. Other experts have brought to the surface that a degree of the susceptibility to breast cancer, from a genetic perspective, might be a result of a breast cancer-susceptibility locus linked to the ABO locus located on specific chromosomes. Basically these experts are saying that you may be able to predict breast cancer according to blood type to some degree.

Health Alert! Lung cancer is one of the leading causes of deaths from cancer in the United States. The incidence of lung cancer has steadily been decreasing in men over the past few years, but interesting is

still on the rise for women. The most common preventable cause is cigarette smoking and second hand smoke, followed by exposure to harmful chemicals in the environment.

Blood Type A and Cancer

Breast Cancer

In general women in blood group A seem to have faster progression of cancer and a worse outcome. Research shows women with group A blood type are the majority of breast cancer cases. This is evident even with women that are believed to be low-risk. One of the most significant risk factors with fast progressing cancer is type A blood.

Female Reproductive Cancers

As a general rule of thumb reproductive cancers are more often found in women with group A blood, and the prognosis is worse. In many reproductive cancers the worse-case scenario with any aspect of it is seen in this blood group.

Bladder Cancer

With this cancer group A doesn't get the short end of the stick. In fact studies have shown people with blood group A have lower death rates and severity of tumors. Group B blood is actually protective of bladder cancer.

Lung Cancer

A higher number of groups A develop lung cancer and an even higher number in the under 50 age group.

Blood Type O and Cancer

Breast Cancer

Women with O blood type are on the complete opposite end of the spectrum here. In fact experts believe type O women have a built in resistance to developing breast cancer. Of the type O women that develop breast cancer, they're significantly less likely to die from it.

Female Reproductive Cancers

Type O blood women seem to have less occurrences of various reproductive cancers and they are more likely to have a better prognosis and outcome.

Type O blood is known to have a better five year survival rate with cervical cancer and ovarian cancer, along with a better five and ten year survival rate for endometrial cancer.

Bladder Cancer

The tables are turned and type O has larger, higher grade and more aggressive bladder cancer. This cancer tends to progress the fastest, result in death more often and replace more frequently.

Lung Cancer

Again group O seems to have a natural protection that deters cells from mutating. If cancer is detected it's generally not as aggressive, lower mortality rate, and less incidence of recurring.

Blood Type AB and Cancer

Breast Cancer

Women with group AB blood steer closer to type A susceptibility to breast cancer. They have a gentle increase in developing it, are more likely to have it recur, and have shorter survival times.

Female Reproductive Cancers

The worse rate of survival is found in the blood group AB, along with type B. This also means the survival rate is the poorest at just five and ten years.

Bladder Cancer

Group AB gets some protection here adapting the natural protection blood group A has against bladder cancer.

Lung Cancer

Group AB seems to stick close with type A blood and has a higher number of lung cancer cases in general. Recurrence is also higher.

Blood Type B and Cancer

Breast Cancer

Research shows women with blood group B tend to be a little closer to group O, with a degree of natural resistance to breast cancer. With women that have no history of it this is even more likely to be true. Keep in mind if you are a woman with group B blood and have a family member with breast cancer, your natural protection isn't valid. In fact you need to take extra precautions to avoid developing breast cancer. If you happen to have battled breast cancer and are group B blood, your odds of recurrence increase drastically.

Female Reproductive Cancers

Group B women fall in closely behind type O blood women in reproductive cancers. They are also less likely to have a malignant tumor of the ovaries. Make the note Type B has a better five year survival rate for ovarian cancer.

Bladder Cancer

Group B tends to be not far from O with regards to bladder cancer. It doesn't have a natural protection against it, occurring more frequently and with a vengeance.

Lung Cancer

Type B mimics O with some protection against lung cancer. With a lower rate of incidence, it doesn't come back as often and the outlook is generally more promising.

It seems to be in general when it comes to cancers, group A has an increased risk for most, faster manifestation, a higher recurrence, high deal rate and greater severity overall. Group AB for the most part leans towards A results, just with a little less severity. Group O tends to consistently have the lowest incidence of cancers in general with a protection naturally in the body. If cancer develops it tends to be less drastic, less likely to recur, shorter in duration and the mortality rate is lower. Type B blood groups are usually closest to type O and also have some natural resistance within the body against most cancers.

The above applies to the following cancer types:

* *Gall Bladder/Live/Pancreatic Cancer*

* *Colon Cancer*

* *Esophagus and Oral Cavity Cancers*

* *Brain Cancers*

* *Thyroid Cancer*

* *Melanoma*

* *Bone Cancers*

My Thinking . . .

There are some things in life that are uncontrollable, two of which are your genetic and blood type. You can sit and pout about your blood type or you can use this information and decide to make better food choices for you that are going to help reflect your health in a more positive light, along with making healthy lifestyle choices and getting your routine checkups. When it comes to cancers any information you have is good information because it's the unknown that's the problem.

Understanding nothing is written in stone and there's always exceptions to the rule. Keep in mind the research findings in regard to specific cancers and blood types, and take the necessary steps to ensure you do everything you can to keep cancer out and in great health.

Water Importance

It's important that you drink quality water and plenty of it for good health. Water is essential for your body biochemical and physiological well-being. This means that regardless of your blood type you need water to function mentally and physically.

Water Facts

* Blood is over 80% water, essential in transporting nutrients to vital organs and internal systems
* Your brain is over 70% water
* Muscles are composed of 75% water
* Lungs pump oxygen and are over 80% water
* Your bones have 25% water

Water is critical in the function of your body, from nerve impulses to breathing, and carrying essential nutrients throughout your body. Not getting enough water can cause dehydration, with symptoms like:

- Headache and extreme fatigue
- Constipation
- Muscle cramping and confusion

PAIN AND DEHYDRATION

I'm guessing you will be able to relate to your body signaling pain because of dehydration. When you don't give your body enough water lactic acid builds up internally in your cells, which would normally be cleared with water. The result may be:

* heartburn or pain from colitis
* back pain or dyspeptic pain
* joint pain

* morning sickness and migraines
* fibromyalgia

What people often miss is that many types of pain are a direct result of dehydration.

My Thoughts . . .

Water is essential to all living organisms. Without water we could not survive. And regardless of the style of eating you choose it's critically important you give your body what it needs, which means plenty of water. Water is going to help all of your internal systems run smoothly, along with giving you the energy and positive mindset you need to live every day to the fullest.

In keeping things basic, make sure regardless you drink 6-8 glasses of water EVERY DAY. Develop this habit and adjust as required and your great health will thank you for it.

Myths and Truths about Diet

Myth - Losing fat fast by dieting is best for permanent weight loss.

Fact - Losing fat quickly with the fad diet of the week is NOT the route to go. Restricting calories generally mean you are missing essential nutrients from your diet. Starving yourself isn't going to work either, which is inevitable with many fad diets. If your daily calorie count dips below 1200, depending on your height, weight, physical composition and exercise schedule, you will trigger your body into starvation mode. It will automatically start storing every carrot stick you eat as fat because your body doesn't trust when you're going to eat again. Your rate in which you burn fat and calories (metabolism) will slow, energy will be almost nonexistent and you are going to feel like crap. That's the basic scenario anyway.

Your best route to lose fat for good is to make healthy food choices, exercise in moderation and adopt the foods that are made for your blood type. It doesn't hurt to try right?

Myth - Foods like celery and grapefruit help you lose weight by burning fat.

Fact - There aren't any specific foods that burn fat. Sure some foods with caffeine may help boost your metabolism for a little while. But this significance really isn't enough to help you lose weight - sorry!

Myth - Carbohydrates make you fat.

Fact - Well this isn't entirely true because too much of any food will make you fat! What many people fail to consider is there are two kinds of carbohydrates: Simple and Complex

Simple carbohydrates are converted to energy quickly by your body but this energy only lasts a short time and is often loaded with fat and calories and few nutrients. Just think white breads, cakes, cookies, chocolate bars, sweets etc. However fruits are considered simple carbohydrates and are an exception to the rule because they are full of natural sugars and contain loads of vitamins and minerals. Too many simple carbohydrates are going to wreak havoc with your blood sugar levels, mood and hormones, interfere with sleep and they will make you fat, particularly if you get into the habit of overdosing.

Complex carbohydrates on the other hand are essential to good health. They take longer to digest, have lots of fiber and will help you sustain your energy levels instead of spiking your energy up and down throughout the day. Examples are healthy whole grains, whole wheat pasta and rice, beans and sweet potatoes.

Glucose that is only found in carbohydrates is needed for your liver, brain, kidneys, muscles and nervous system to function. If you don't get your best carbs you can end up with kidney and liver damage, along with hallucinations to start.

So make sure you get the carbs you need each day. Just keep it in moderation and stay away from the junky fat ones!

Myth - Choosing no-fat or low-fat equates to no calories.

Fact - You need to be very careful here because although no fat is usually lower in fat than the "normal" version, many of them have just as many calories. As well they might usually have sugar, extra fillers and unnatural thickeners to make them taste and look better. Of course this is adding extra calories for all the wrong reasons.

Just make sure you check the label and know how much fat and how many calories are in something before you toss it in your basket. It's a learning process I know but you've got to start somewhere.

Myth - Fast foods are always an unhealthy choice.

Fact - For the most part fast foods are best left alone. However attention has recently been heightened in regards to worldly healthy eating and this has forced those infamous fast food joints to step up to the plate. Most now offer healthy alternatives that aren't "awesome," but can still be okay to indulge in from time to time. Ordering a greasy burger, large fries and supersized shake is definitely not going to help your belt cinch tighter. But, by moderating your eating and making a few adjustments you can enjoy fast food and not get fat over it.

Try looking for healthy items like grilled chicken salad with dressing on the side, or a grilled small burger on a whole wheat bun, easy on the condiments. If you REALLY need to have some fries just order the kiddy size or share with a friend, while you're filling your belly full with your tasty grilled chicken salad. It's all about give and take here and knowing that when eating fast food today, you do have an opportunity to make healthier food choices. It's you that's in control of you though.

Myth - Eating anytime after 8 is going to make you gain weight.

Fact - That's hogwash! What you need to look at is what you eat and how much you eat over a period of time. It's easiest to break your eating time frames into days. For instance, the average women of normal size and moderate exercise level needs about 2200 calories a day to maintain her weight. So it really doesn't matter when she gets theses calories throughout the day in order to maintain her weight.

What makes sense though is that you eat your nutritious food regularly throughout the day in small amounts. This will help you keep your blood sugars level and energy always available when you need it. You don't need to eat a gigantic meal at 7 pm because your body will soon be shutting down for the night. Make the smart choice to eat a little more at breakfast time and then evenly throughout the day. If anything you should eat a little less later on, not unless you plan on doing an aerobics session in your sleep!

Myth - Red meat is bad for you and will interfere with losing weight.

Your body needs protein to energize you, build lean muscle and keep your mind crisp and sharp, to start anyway. Protein is a macronutrient which means your body needs lots of it. Protein isn't manufactured by your body and it really can't be stored. This means you need to consume it in small amounts regularly in order to stay healthy and happy. Meat is the best route to do this because it is what we call a complete protein, as opposed to incomplete proteins found in numerous other foods like beans and vegetables. Red meat, pork, chicken and fish also have lots of other vitamins and minerals your body needs. The key is moderation and choosing lean cuts of meat because you don't need the added cholesterol and unhealthy fat many meats offer.

Myth - If you are a vegetarian this means you are healthier and will lose weight.

Fact - On average, people eating vegetarian consume fewer calories because of the food choices they make. So it makes sense they tend to weigh less than those of us that are meat eaters. This doesn't mean that vegetarians can't be fat and unhealthy. Too much of anything isn't a good thing and if vegetarians choose to eat lots of high-fat, high-calorie foods that don't have any nutritional value, they will become unhealthy and heavier.

In other words, it's important you make healthy food choices and eat them in moderation if you are looking to get healthy and lean, regardless of the "type" of eating your choice.

My Thinking . . .

You only know what you know. What's important is that you gain knowledge by separating fact from fiction because you're only going to better your health and wellness decisions if you have the correct information to start.

Final Thoughts

Information is knowledge and knowledge is power. The more you learn about your body and how it works, the better you'll be able to figure out what sort of foods work best for getting you to your optimal level of health and wellness. It's not about a quick-fix here. Your health is important and this means you need to have patience and take the time to implement the changes one at a time that are going to get you healthier and happier with a smile.

If you truly hate the changes you are trying to make then you shouldn't make them. Through trial and error you will figure out your tolerance and preferences and slowly but surely you will fit the puzzle pieces together that gives you the body you've always wanted, energy levels to match, and a positive outlook on life in general because you know you are taking the steps necessary to take care of you; mind, body and soul.

Eating right for your blood type is just one more piece of knowledge you can use to help determine which fuel sources and in what amounts are right for you. The ones that are going to help deter disease from setting in, help you build lean muscle and zap fat, sharpen your thinking, and leave you looking and feeling like a million bucks. You are unique and so should be your healthy eating. My hope is that you have gained new knowledge from the blood eating diet perspective and can use it positively towards your good health.

Good Luck!

We have the choice to look for the positive or the negative in life. You can choose to lift someone up or to stomp on them. Writing is my passion and I work hard at it, with the goal of helping make people better. If you gain a new piece of knowledge, read something that makes you think, or perhaps even smile a few times, then I am happy and content!

Life's just too short not to tune into optimism. If your glass is half full, then I invite you to read my writing, and if you have a minute to spare when you're through, **I would appreciate your review.** This will help me better myself and my writing. I thank you in advance and appreciate you.

CPSIA information can be obtained at www.ICGtesting.com
Printed in the USA
LVOW05s1939070414

380676LV00037B/1979/P

9 781493 766062